R.E.I. Editions

All of our ebooks can be read on the following devices:
- Computers
- eReaders
- iOS
- Android
- Blackberries
- Windows
- Tablet
- Cell phone

French Academy

Muladhara

The First chakra

ISBN: 978-2-37297-3540

Publication: January 2019
New updated edition: January 2023
Copyright © 2019 - 2023 R.E.I. Editions
www.rei-editions.com

Work plan

French Academy

Muladhara
The First Chakra

R.E.I. Editions

Book Index

The chakra system

The word Chakra, which comes from Sanskrit and means "wheel", is meant to indicate the seven basic energy centers in the human body. Chakras are centers of subtle psychic energy located along the spine. Each of these centers is connected, at the level of subtle energies, to the main ganglia of the nerves which branch off from the vertebral column. In addition, the chakras are related to the levels of consciousness, to the archetypal elements, to the phases inherent in the development of life, to the colors, which are closely linked to the chakras, because they are found outside our body, but inside the aura , or the electromagnetic field that surrounds each person, to sounds, body functions and much, much more. The Eastern doctrine that has spread knowledge of them in the Western world considers the Chakras as openings, gateways to the essence of the human body. The chakras are usually represented inside a lotus flower, with a variable number of open petals. The open petals represent the chakra in its full opening. On each petal is written one of the fifty letters of the Sanskrit alphabet, which are considered sacred letters, therefore, divine expression. Furthermore, each of them expresses a different activity of the human being, a different state, both manifest and still potential. Each chakra resonates on a different frequency which corresponds to the colors of the rainbow.

The seven main Chakras also correspond to the seven main glands of our endocrine system. Their main function is to absorb the Universal Energy, metabolize it, break it down and convey it along the energy channels up to the nervous system, feed the auras and release energy outside. Most everyone sees them as funnels, simultaneously swirling and flowing energy back and forth. Each of the seven centers has both an anterior (usually dominant) component and a posterior (usually less dominant) component, which are intimately connected, with the exception, however, of the first and seventh, which, however, are single.

From the second to the fifth, the anterior aspect relates to feelings and emotions, while the posterior aspect relates to the will. As regards the anterior and posterior sixth, and the seventh, the correlation is with the mind and reason. The first and seventh. they also have the very important connection function for the human being: being the most external Chakras of the energy channel, they have the characteristic of placing man in relation with the Universe on one side and with the Earth on the other. The perfect functioning of the energy system is synonymous with good health. There are many techniques to open the Chakras, including Reiki, which stands out for its peculiar sweetness and for the possibility of harmonizing any energy imbalances.

Each center oversees certain organs, and has particular functions on an emotional, psychic and spiritual level. Among the seven fundamental ones, there are precise affinities.

- The First with the Seventh: Basic Energy with Spirit Energy.
- The Second with the Sixth: Energy of feeling on a material level with Energy of feeling on an extrasensory level.
- The Third with the Fifth: Energy of the working mind and personal power with Energy of the higher mind and communication.
- The Fourth: bridge between the upper three and the lower three and alchemical forge of transformation.

Each Chakra is associated with a color, which corresponds to and derives from the frequency and vibration of the center itself. Furthermore, each Chakra corresponds to a mantra, the sound of a musical note and, in some cases, even a natural element, a planet or a zodiac sign. Because the chakra system is the primary processing center for every function of our being, blockage or energetic insufficiency in the chakras usually causes unrest in body, mind, or spirit. A defect in the flow of energy through a given chakra will cause a defect in the energy supplied to the connected parts of the physical body, as well as affect all levels of being. This is because an energy field is a Holistic entity; every part of it affects every other part. Essential oils are able to tune into specific chakras: their scent and their vibration gently put us in deep contact with our energy centers.

The massage with specific essential oils on the points corresponding to the chakras activates and balances their action, harmonizing and strengthening the entire body. Starting from the bottom they are:

- 1st = Muladhara
- 2nd = Swadhisthana
- 3rd = Manipura
- 4th = Anahata
- 5th = Vhishuddhi
- 6th = Ajna
- 7th = Sahasrara

Furthermore, each of the seven chakras comes to represent an important area of human psychic health, which we can briefly summarize as:

1. Survival
2. Sexuality
3. Strength
4. Love
5. Communication
6. Intuition
7. Cognition.

Metaphorically the chakras are related to the following archetypal elements:

1. Earth
2. Water
3. Fire
4. Air
5. Sound
6. Light
7. Thought

Muladhara - The First Chakra

The first chakra is called the "base chakra" or "root chakra" and is therefore connected with earthly existence on a purely physical level and with smell. It is the first of the seven energy centers of our body and is located at the base of the spine, in the perineum area, between the genitals and the anus. It is the first Chakra starting from the bottom and this position makes it the support of all the others. Its symbol is the red lotus with four petals inscribed in gold with the last four consonants of the Sanskrit alphabet: «v, sh (lingual), sh (palatal), s». Muladhara is a single vortex pointing downwards towards the earth, it has no front or back movement like the other chakras. From here originate the three energy channels Sushumna, Ida and Pingala. Its functioning harmonizes with the seventh chakra, therefore, with the hypothalamic-pituitary-gonad-adrenal neuro-hormonal axis. Through this energy center the knowledge stored in the collective unconscious manifests itself. The Muladhara chakra constitutes the foundation and root of the chakra energy system, as through it the energy emanating from the earth and nature is collected and subsequently transformed. It is, therefore, the foundation of the other chakras, it is the earth in which to anchor the roots and give stability, security and defense. Its main function is survival and the associated keyword: "I exist".

It is oriented vertically with the funnel opening towards the Earth. Its main function would be linked to the material body, to the survival instinct and would produce a sense of physical and mental harmony in relation to nature, satisfying primordial needs such as food, water, air, rest.

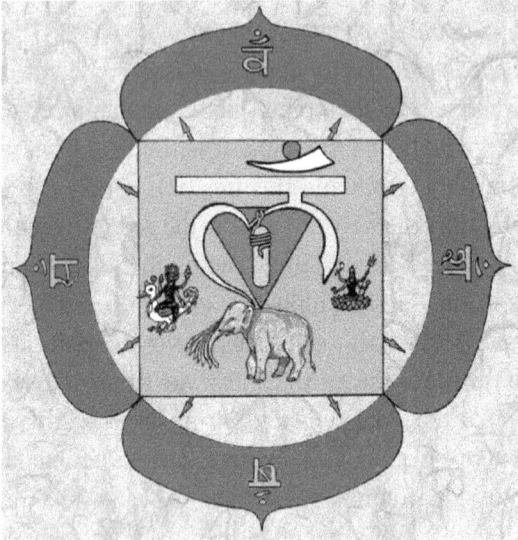

The first chakra, since it has only one pole, would tend to be a bit larger than the other chakras. Its geometric symbol is the triangle with a vertex at the bottom enclosed in a square, the first emblems of the female sexual organ and the second of the Earth element; in it sleeps Kundalini. In the Traipura triangle, whose three sides are presided over by the female deities Vama, Jyeshtha and Raudri, personifications of will, knowledge and action, resides the goddess Tripurasundari in the form of her bijamantra «klim». Also within the triangle is the lingam Svayamhhu, splendid as molten gold and in the shape of a bud wrapped around itself, radiating lunar splendor, seat of Shiva with a green-blue complexion. The mouth of the lingam, the Brahmadvara, or the "Gate of Brahma", is blocked by Kundalini, coiled like a snake three and a half times on itself, dazzling like a thunderbolt and softly "buzzing" like a swarm of bees. Lady of beings, enchantress, source of sound, she confuses the world with her illusory games and only the yogi manages to dispel her veils. Kundalini is described as a splendid young woman seated on a lion, with three eyes and four arms with two hands in a gesture that dispels fear (hand raised with palm visible), and bestows gifts (hand lowered with palm always visible), while holding in the other two a book and a lute. The divinity in charge of this wheel is Brahma, her vital energy takes the name of Savitri or bride of the creator. The sense organ related to the muladhara is the nose, seat of smell, while the organ of action are the feet, in direct contact with the earth, anchored to it by the force of gravity but at the same time the base that allows the body to get up and stretch upwards. The main characteristic of this chakra is hardness, so the concentration on mooladhara favors strengthening and stability.

The bjamantra is «lam», that is the Sanskrit letter «la» nasalized, that is pronounced making it resonate in the nose. It is the bijamantra of the god Indra, lord of the gods in the most ancient period of Hindu civilization, the one centered on the sacred collections of the Vedas. The bijamantra is visualized as a four-armed divinity, of golden yellow color, on the back of the elephant

Airavata, the mount of Indra, in some later representations represented black. "Lam" is also the bijamantra of Dhara, the earth goddess. Another divinity is inscribed in the dot placed on the letter of the Sanskrit alphabet to nasalize it, the god Brahma, lord of the origin of the universe, endowed with four faces and represented here as a child. His mount is the white goose with a striped head, an animal that in the Hindu tradition represents the soul and which is identified with the swan by Western translators. Shakti, the feminine cosmic energy, is projected here as Dakini, a terrifying goddess on a red lotus that opens inside the main flower: this additional lotus underlines with its bright color the powerful and yet to be controlled energy of nature . Dakini, resplendent like the rising sun, dressed in black, with a fierce face and red eyes, has four arms in whose hands are the spear, the khatvanga (a stick with a skull stuck on it), the sword and the cup filled with intoxicating liquid . Dakini purifies the intellect and bestows enlightenment. She is fond of rice pudding, sugar and milk and is associated with plasma, one of the seven tissues that traditional Indian medicine, Ayurveda, believes to make up the human body. The first is the chakra of the beginning of growth and it is not possible to avoid exploring it thoroughly, accepting it and illuminating it if you want to start a path of growth and spiritual evolution. It would be connected to the kidneys and adrenal glands.

Its physiological functions would concern the production of blood and bones and reproductive activities. An "earth energy" would arrive from this chakra and its closing would produce the sensation that "the earth is missing under your feet". In Greek mythology it is said that man was created from clay and that our mother is Gea, the Earth. The first chakra indicates how the person is at that moment with respect to his physical energies. If the person is happy to live, if he is in good health, at least if he believes he has a good relationship with his body, if he wants to have fun, to play. This Chakra is normally associated with the adrenal glands, lower limbs, spine, large intestine, genitals, and central nervous system. It develops from the moment of birth to the completion of the first 24 months of life, allowing the child to grow physically and to develop motor skills. The Root Chakra has a strong influence on one's career and relationship with money. Its proper functioning affects professional life, financial balance and one's sense of belonging. If there is excessive functioning of this Chakra, both thoughts and actions will be oriented towards the obsessive satisfaction of material needs and personal safety; you will want to possess everything you want, while it will be difficult to give or donate anything. If hindered, one reacts with aggression, anger, violence, feelings or methods that express a defensive attitude, linked to the lack of trust in the ancestral vital forces; in this attitude there is always the fear of losing what gives security and a sense of well-being.

If, on the other hand, there is insufficient functionality, there will be weakness and poor physical and emotional resistance. Many things will be lived with excessive concern, even if they are very trivial. Existential insecurity, in the meaning most linked to primordial instincts, will be the main problem, you will feel as if you have lost all footholds. Every fact of life will become insurmountable, therefore easier, more pleasant and less tiring conditions will be dreamed of, generating mental escapes from contingent reality. If the upper Chakras have developed more than the lower ones, one will have the feeling of being out of the world, deeply experiencing a sense of estrangement and absolute and hopeless loneliness. If the energy block also affects the third Chakra, in addition to the first, one could find oneself in the presence of anorexia. The pathologies that can cause its disharmonious functioning are due to:

- Physical complaints, such as bowel disease, constipation, hemorrhoids, sciatic nerve disorders, back pain, varicose veins, bladder and kidney disorders, prostate pain, bone disease, anemia, blood pressure fluctuations.
- Mental disorders, such as phobias, weakness, depression, lack of confidence, tendency to depend too much on others.

The sense of the first chakra is smell, the first sense that the newborn actively uses. Animals are recognized primarily through smell; they know how to recognize the smell of fear (the adrenaline that escapes from the pores when we "sweat cold"). This is why dogs know who is afraid. Adrenaline causes blood vessels to constrict, thereby increasing blood pressure. The effect is twofold: a greater quantity of blood nourishes the muscles but blocks the digestive functions. The use of perfumes indicates that smell is an important sense. However, those who are in good health and who follow the right diet do not need deodorants or perfumes, because they will already have a pleasant and attractive smell. Smell receptors are located at the base of the brain and feed directly into the limbic system, which is the area of memory and emotion. Therefore, aromas can immediately access emotional memories that are found in our unconscious. The animal of the first chakra is the elephant with seven trunks. In Europe too, the elephant suggests primordial strength: it knows how to stay in a group and knows how to die alone. We appreciate this animal's intellect because it remembers its benefactors (as well as its enemies) and is gentle: it only eats vegetables and knows its own strength, it will never crush a living being. The representation with seven proboscis seems curious: it symbolizes the seven aspects of the whole life and of each specific period, the seven types of energy that are available during the day, in short, the seven chakras.

Each chakra supplies prana to a different endocrine gland. Just as there are seven chakras, there are seven endocrine glands. Both the chakras and the endocrine glands are located along the spinal column.

- The endocrine glands produce hormones and supply them to the bloodstream. These glands lack an excretory duct, therefore, the hormones are released directly into the bloodstream where they are carried to every organ and tissue by the blood to exert their influence on all functions of the physical body.

Each gland is internally related to other glands and also works closely with the nervous and circulatory systems. In order for the organs of the body to function efficiently, the blood must contain certain chemicals and these chemicals are secreted by the endocrine glands. The secretion of the glands into the endocrine system is vital to the health of the entire system. Our bodies can get sick if there are too few or too many hormones. The endocrine glands of the first chakra are the adrenal glands. There are two adrenal glands located above the top of each of the two kidneys. The adrenal glands are the body's call to battle. When adrenaline is released into the system, our perceptions become clearer, we have new vigor and feel more courageous. The release of adrenaline activates the fight/flight syndrome, which prepares us for battle or flight. The release of adrenaline and the activation of fight/flight are generated by real or imagined dangers. Thus, our emotions can trigger an adrenaline release when we feel extreme fear or even chronic anxiety. The first chakra is the "survival chakra" and the fight/flight syndrome is vital to the survival of the species. According to the doctrine of Yoga, the energy of the Kundalini (sexual energy) resides in this chakra: if the base is stable, the energy can ascend through the other chakras thus accelerating the development of the personality. As mentioned, the First Chakra is the main generator of the human energy system and is connected with all solid things that exist on earth, primarily the body and the satisfaction of essential needs. The subjects focused in

Muladhara are very strong and resistant people, endowed with a concrete temperament, oriented towards the simple satisfaction of material needs. They have a slow and limited mind, but effective for everything related to the relationship with material objects or the ability to survive and the task of obtaining the necessary.

They usually choose jobs that require a lot of muscle strength, or related to the production of solid and resistant objects, or repetitive jobs. In cases where the Chakra is fairly balanced, they also prove to be very constant people, with very little imagination and a great attachment to traditions, family habits and place of birth.

- Chakra in a state of lightness: it is the enlightened condition of the Chakra, in which the capacities for concreteness that are typical of this center are placed at the service of an idea and a purpose. Subjects with an almost infinite patience. It also develops a proper attention to the body and its health.

- Chakra in a dynamic state: it is marked by a great energy which is applied in work and in the production of objects, in building and in accumulating material goods. Instinct for hunting and fighting. If there is a strong excess of Rajas, it will give rise to action aimed at accumulation, difficulties in relationships due to excessive attachment and pettiness, dispersive and meaningless acting, highly destructive impulses.

- Chakra in a state of heaviness: heaviness is the quality of the energy that naturally dominates this Chakra. If a further excess of Tamas develops, a state of inertia, dullness, laziness, drowsiness, brutality and unconsciousness is created. Nutrition, aerobic movement, regular practice of Asana and Pranayama and positive mental stimuli are the best way out of this dangerous and obscure condition, which can block evolution and push the individual towards very low and degenerates.

How to activate the 1st chakra

- To harmonize the first chakra, the body must be trained and exercise constantly. Gym, long walks, go for a run.

- Gain awareness of your feet and legs by going for walks in the woods or mountains and applying jets of cold water to your thighs.

- Seek a link with the earth, staying as immersed in nature as possible and working as much as possible in the garden.

- Allow yourself a short massage every day in the logical reflex zones of your feet.

- The vowel "U" stimulates the first chakra, sit upright, inhale through the nose and make the "U" resonate while exhaling, performing this exercise for 5 minutes.

- Use connected stones.

Color of the first chakra

The energy of colors acts on the chakras at the level of clothes worn, food ingested and presence in the environment in which we live. Learning to know and use them helps us to find psycho-physical harmony in a respectful and non-invasive way. Chromotherapy has an effect on the brain through the hypothalamus, which regulates and controls the endocrine glands, and therefore also the energy centers of man, associated with the autonomic nervous system and with the regulation of hormones. The spectrum of the seven colors of the rainbow, or of the light reflected through a prism, corresponds to that of the scale of the seven chakras, from the lowest to the highest.

- Red is the color of the first chakra.

Wear red clothing or use red fabrics in your home, put red roses on your table. Complementary colors are black, gray and brown. Red is the color of the earth, of blood, of physicality, the rainbow begins its spectrum with the color red. The word red in Latin is indicated with the terms "rutilus and ruber" which conceptually mean "blood and life"; red is the symbol of the body, of matter. This is a color that remains firm on itself, it does not radiate outside or inside itself. Whoever chooses this color, in light form denotes security, self-confidence, harmony with one's body, joy. In the shadow form it denotes the need to be gratified, the overestimation of oneself, one is childish.

This is the color of love but also of war and death, it is a great energy activator. In alchemy it represents the sun, man, sulfur and gold, for the American Indians it indicates fertility, life, the ancient Egyptians used it to protect themselves from fire. Nowadays we have red fire extinguishers and fire engines, in ancient times warriors and hunters used to paint and decorate their bodies with the color red, for them it meant strength and protection. A natural dye for dyeing fabrics is extracted from madder root. This color was obtained from molluscs (murici), the operation was long and expensive for this in antiquity, red represented power and wealth (Purple); in the beginning it was used exclusively by the religious, later it was also used by the sovereigns. Red represents a physiological condition of stimulus and excitement. Its effects on the psyche are of strong physical energy, the energy of red acts on sexuality and survival instinct. As foods, prefer red colored foods (apples and beets), hot spices (red pepper, cayenne pepper, tabasco), earthy vegetables (potatoes and carrots), animal proteins (red meat and eggs).

Essential oils associated with the first chakra

Sandalwood, Patchouli, Cedarwood, Incense, Sage, Vetiver, Cloves, Ginger, Benzoin. Mix each individual essential oil with a carrier oil, such as jojoba or almond oil, in the ratio of 2 drops per tablespoon of carrier oil, i.e., 2 drops per 10 mL of carrier. Since this is a "vibrational treatment", a very diluted mixture will have a deeper and more marked action. Massage the chakra you want to work on with the blend containing the chosen essential oil. Use a few drops and apply them slowly with your fingertips and in a clockwise circular motion. In the case of this first chakra, the sole of the foot or the tip of the coccyx can be massaged. While massaging the Chakra, focus on the result you want to achieve, visualizing the harmonic energy of the oil as it opens and rebalances the chakra. After the treatment, lie down and relax for a while, allowing the Chakra to rebalance itself. Breathe deeply and slowly, trying to clear and empty your mind as much as possible. As an alternative to the massage, add a few drops of the essential oil chosen for the treatment to the essence diffuser. Concentrate and focus on your therapeutic intention, visualize the aromatherapy energy of the essential oil, open and rebalance the chakra. Relax for at least half an hour.

Sandalwood

For 4,000 years the aroma of sandalwood essential oil has been appreciated, so much so that it is traditionally used in Tantric Yoga schools to help awaken Kundalini, sexual energy. One of the properties of sandalwood oil is that it improves over time, i.e. it matures particular notes that make it even more pleasant. Unfortunately, the inconsiderate use of these trees for the vast production of oils both for curative purposes and for the production of soaps and perfumes, has caused a drastic decrease in the number of specimens which are now monitored to prevent their disappearance. On a physical level, sandalwood is one of the most delicate essential oils for the skin: it does not irritate, restores the right hydration and heals small wounds. Due to its antiseptic and decongestant properties it is a panacea for respiratory tract problems.

1. Part used - wood and roots.
2. Extraction method - steam distillation.
3. Base note: woody, sweet, balsamic, intense scent.

- **Aphrodisiac**

Transform sexual energy by elevating it to the spiritual plane. It reduces aggression and violent instincts, loosens exasperation and releases blocked sexual energy. Sexual disorders related to depressive states are often resolved thanks to the use of this oil. It is, however, more suitable for active people than for phlegmatic subjects. Although it has always been considered a powerful and precise signal of male eros, sandalwood essential oil gives off a soft and warm force that envelops men and women with equal beneficial effects. It works by balancing sexuality with the spirit, promoting the integration of the sacred with the profane: for this reason it is used in tantra yoga schools to transform sexual energies into spiritual energies. It is therefore not a direct aphrodisiac, as its action is predominantly meditative and directed towards the interiority: it is indicated for subjects who experience sexuality in a superficial way.

- **Harmonizing**

Sandalwood essential oil balances the entire chakra energy system by calming and facilitating spiritual development. Its particular value consists in the fact that it manages to calm the mental work that often distracts those who meditate. By stilling the rational part of the mind, it allows it to enter the deeper stages of meditation. This is advisable when preparing to take a healing session and in self-healing. Transmits openness of mind, warmth and understanding. Reduces stress, calms aggression, agitation and fear, indicated in case of insomnia. It supports those who practice yoga against anxiety and depression, to find serenity.

- **Relaxing bath**

10 drops of essential oil in bath water give a pleasant feeling of relaxation. Remain immersed for at least 15 minutes. Some parents greatly appreciate the scent of sandalwood essential oil diluted in a base oil or in the bathtub in case of problems with hyperactive, stubborn children or to calm rebellious teenagers.

- **Shower**

Put 3-4 drops on a wet sponge glove and gently massage the whole body.

- **Contraindications**

Sandalwood essential oil is non-irritating, non-sensitizing and non-toxic. It is good to pay attention not to use it in case of severe kidney disease and for periods not exceeding 6 weeks. Contraindicated in pregnancy and breastfeeding. Particular caution is required at the time of purchase as it is often "cut" with lower quality essences, such as, for example, the essential oil of Australian sandalwood.

Patchouli

The scent of patchouli evokes the refuge of deep and humid woods, arousing in those who inhale it the feeling of intimacy with themselves. He has a toning and stimulating action useful in case of depression and mental torpor; while it is calming and relaxing in case of anxiety and stress.

In aromatherapy it is indicated for young people, who find it difficult to identify with their bodies and allows those who live in an exalted dimension of mental and psychic experiences to remain grounded. In these properties lies the explanation of the fascination it has always had on the new generations, who all have in common two attributes of the adolescent and pre-adult phase: the physical arrogance of hormonal momentum and great idealistic aspirations. Patchouli allows you to harmoniously reconcile them. Patchouli essential oil is not only the aroma of youth, but also has beneficial antidepressant effects on adults who, due to their social life and professional life, have to control their physical impulses, and suffer from psycho-physical exhaustion, anxiety or sexual disorders.

It has a euphoric effect on these people, because it induces the pituitary gland to produce endorphins, the feel-good hormone. To calm anxious states, put 12 drops of Patchouli essential oil in 200 ml of water. With a cloth, make compresses on the forehead and temples.

Also wet your wrists and lie down in the dark, changing the compresses from time to time.

Also put a few drops of this essence in the special burner placing it in the room where you lie down.

As an aphrodisiac, it induces the pituitary gland to produce endorphins (euphoric) useful for those who cannot let go (frigidity) or have a decrease in libido: it increases concentration and energy. Recommended for more mature people who, due to their social life and professional life, have to control their physical urges, and suffer from psycho-physical exhaustion or sexual disorders.

1. Part used: leaves.
2. Method of extraction: steam distillation.
3. Base note: intense and persistent aroma, earthy, sour, sweet and spicy.

- **Aphrodisiac**

Induces the pituitary gland to produce endorphins (euphoric) useful for those who cannot let go (frigidity) or have a decrease in libido: it increases concentration and energy. Recommended for more mature people who, due to their social life and professional life, have to control their physical urges, and suffer from psycho-physical exhaustion or sexual disorders.

- **Relaxing bath**

Put 10 drops in the bath water; immerse yourself for 10 minutes, against states of anxiety and stress. When we get out of the tub, the beneficial effects of patchouli will also be visible on the skin: the skin will appear more toned and luminous.

- **Healing**

In massage oil, it has a repairing action on the skin tissue, counteracting the formation of stretch marks and wrinkles: useful in case of dry, tired and aged skin, and in disorders such as dermatitis, acne, cracks and burns.

- **Contraindications**

Contraindicated for internal use, during pregnancy and lactation. At the recommended doses, it has no contraindications. Do not administer to children.

Cedar wood

Since ancient times, it has always been a highly sought-after tree for its precious wood, rich in essential oil, widely used to build houses, because the aroma it gave off acted as a repellent for insects. In Egypt it was used, together with other essential oils, during the embalming ritual to block the processes of putrefaction and to preserve the papyri from parasitic destruction. The oil, extracted by steam distillation from the bark or sawdust of the red cedar, was perhaps the first oil to be extracted. King Solomon's temple was built with the famous cedars of Lebanon, very rare today, and even the American Indians knew it and considered it sacred. They burned it, inhaling its fumes, because it freed the cavities, relaxed the larynx and soothed the soul. The essential oil is a pale yellow-orange liquid, with a sweet and very intense scent, similar to that of camphor with a woody, soft and balsamic note.

Cedarwood essential oil promotes grounding, helps rebalance the first Muladhara chakra and allows you to "focus" on yourself, giving courage, energy, dignity and promoting self-esteem. Particularly useful in times of major changes to manage, such as relocation, removals, change of job; or at the beginning of a new couple relationship it helps not to destabilize too much and not to lose the goal.

The cedar tree, majestic, full of strength and vigor when inhaled, favors the same qualities; it makes fickle, immature and not very determined people stable and determined, it helps to gain respect from others, and to convince without contrasts.

1. Part used: wood from the trunk and branches.
2. Method of extraction: steam distillation.
3. Base note: warm, intense, balsamic, woody, sweet scent.

- **Contraindications**

Internal use is not recommended. Cedarwood essence is contraindicated for children, pregnant and breastfeeding women. It absolutely cannot be ingested, on pain of digestive tract disturbances, nausea and vomiting.

Incense

The Egyptians had introduced incense in their fumigation practices and for cosmetic use: rejuvenating masks and for the preparation of kohl, a sort of kajal for eye make-up. The Jews met it during their stay along the coasts of the Red Sea and included it in their religious practices: connected to the birth of Jesus, brought to him as a gift by the Magi. Even among the Arab peoples, incense was widely used and constituted an exchange wealth. It was also called Olibanum (white). The most valuable variety is, in fact, represented by white grains. The most precious Frankincense essential oil grows at an altitude of 700 meters and comes from Dhofar (Yemen). The tree is engraved in the bark, from which a milky liquid comes out which, in contact with the air, thickens and turns brown, orange, yellow, white, moon drops, with grains almost as large as a walnut ; the grains are selected by the women who separate the delicates from the moonlight color, these give the best quality incense.

- **Aromatherapy**

It is used as a sedative to relieve nervousness, anxiety, black mood, gives courage and confidence. It can be used in the diffuser for meditations. Tonic and rebalancing of the central nervous system, calms anxious forms, stress agitations, obsessive thoughts, fears. In fact, it prepares for calm, meditation and prayer. Against sadness and negative moods, spread 3 or 4 drops of essential oil in the environment; alternatively, take a hot bath by diffusing 5 or 6 drops of essence into the water.

To deeply relax, it will be very useful to perform a light massage on the forehead and temples with 2-3 drops of incense essential oil diluted in 1 tablespoon of vegetable oil.

1. Part used: rubber resin.
2. Method of extraction: steam distillation.
3. Base note: sweet, balsamic scent.

Its perfume is particularly suitable for meditation as it has the property of joining matter to the subtle world of the spirit. It is the purifier par excellence, stimulates mental activity and calms tormented feelings.

- **Bath**

Pour 5 or 6 drops of essential oil into the bathtub, add it to a few drops of eucalyptus and soak for at least 10/15 minutes. In the presence of colds or flu with persistent cough, 6 drops of incense essential oil and 6 of cypress oil will be added to the hot water for the bath mixed in a spoonful of whole honey.

- **Contraindications**

They are not reported against particular indications, except for internal use, as for all essential oils which

must be used with caution and always conveyed; for example, honey is an excellent carrier of essential oils.
A curiosity instead linked to the aroma of incense: it seems that it dampens sexual desire, perhaps incompatible with its strong spiritual value.

Sage

In ancient times, it was considered a sacred plant. Its name derives from the Latin, salvere, from which "to save", because it is believed to be beneficial for any evil. In the Middle Ages it was customary to put a few leaves, rich in essential oil, in the mouth, before going to sleep, to encourage divining dreams or problem solving. In fact, one of the names with which sage was defined in ancient times was "clear eye". It was supposed, in fact, that it strengthened sight and the inner gaze: that it helped to "see" more clearly. Its use in popular tradition was limited to digestive problems, female disorders and nervous disorders, such as anxiety, panic attacks and insomnia, as well as a disinfectant of ulcers and to calm inflammation of the respiratory tract and throat .

1. Part used: flowering tops and leaves.
2. Method of extraction: steam distillation.
3. Heart note: sweet, herbaceous, aromatic scent.

- **Relaxing**

If inhaled, it induces calm and serenity in the presence of stress, nervousness, anguish, fears and paranoia. Excellent support to overcome midlife crises and menopause, for people who no longer dare, the resigned, who feel "too old" and live in a state of depression.

It acts on an emotional level, on our creativity, allowing us to express ourselves and "poetic license" worthy of born artists; instills courage to carry out creative projects or take exams. In case of depression, take 1 drop of essential oil of clary sage and 1 of peppermint in a teaspoon of honey (or a sugar cube) twice a day.

- **Purifying**

Assumed in 2 drops in a teaspoon of honey, it has detoxifying properties on the liver and kidneys, also useful for treating intermittent fevers caused by intestinal infections, poisoning and diarrhea.

- **Healing**

On the skin it has an anti-inflammatory, antimicrobial action and repairs the skin tissue. It is indicated in case of canker sores, dermatitis, sores, insect bites, skin ulcers, acne, fungal infections such as mycosis and candidiasis.

- **Environmental diffusion**

1 drop of sage essential oil for each square meter of the environment in which it spreads, by means of an essential oil burner, or in radiator humidifiers.

- **Contraindications**

Contrary to the "officinal" variety it does not irritate, it does not give sensitization and it is not toxic, but taken in high doses it causes drowsiness, paralysis and convulsions; it is contraindicated in pregnancy and breastfeeding. It is not recommended to use it in conjunction with iron-based medicines or substances and not to associate it with the intake of alcoholic beverages, as it can enhance the effects of alcohol.

Vetiver

The fragrance of vetiver essential oil is as energetic as it is relaxing, and has sedative, toning and aphrodisiac effects. In aromatherapy, due to its multiple properties, this essence is recommended for the treatment of the most diverse ailments. Thanks to its sedative action, vetiver essential oil counteracts nervousness and tension, and is excellent for relaxing the body and mind with a relaxing bath or massage, as well as in the treatment of insomnia.

The simultaneous calming and energizing action makes it very effective in anxious and depressive states, and to counteract psychological tiredness. The toning activity of vetiver essential oil strengthens our body, especially the immune system, stimulates circulation and is effective in counteracting degenerative processes. Vetiver roots are an ancient remedy used in Ayurvedic tradition to relieve headaches and lower fever. In the East the roots were used to create baskets and mats and then sprinkled with water so that on days of great heat they gave off the aroma of vetiver, with insect repellent properties. Vetiver essential oil is obtained by steam distillation of the dried roots of the plant. Base note, this essence shows a certain viscosity and an amber color, and tickles the nose with its sweet and fresh exotic fragrance, with earthy, woody and slightly smoky tones, which recalls the smell of the undergrowth.

In addition to being used alone, vetiver essential oil can be combined with other oils; it goes particularly well with the essences of lavender, yarrow, rose and sage, but also with other base notes such as patchouli and sandalwood.

1. Part used: the dried roots.
2. Method of extraction: steam distillation.
3. Base note: bittersweet, woody, earthy scent

- **Environmental diffusion**

Add 1 drop of vetiver essential oil per square meter of room surface to the diffuser. This will make our home pleasantly scented, giving us purified air and counteracting tension and nervousness.

- **Relaxing bath**

To eliminate anxiety and stress, dilute 15 drops of vetiver essential oil in the tub.

For an even more relaxing effect, immediately after bathing, perform a light massage on the temples and forehead with 2 drops of vetiver essential oil diluted in 1 tablespoon of almond oil.

Shower: 3-4 drops on a wet sponge glove gently massage the whole body.

- **For massage**

2 drops of essential oil to be mixed with an arnica ointment to be applied to soothe joint and muscle pain. Alternatively 3 drops of Vetiver to add to a spoonful of Sesame oil to be massaged on painful areas, or on the abdomen to facilitate digestion.

- **Contraindications**

To be taken externally only. The essential oil must not be used pure directly on the skin or mucous membranes, because it could cause irritation.
Contraindicated during pregnancy and lactation, and in childhood.

Carnation

Since it is an excellent heat stimulant, clove essential oil is also known for its ability to stimulate blood circulation and to help combat feelings of exhaustion. The buds of its dried flowers are the "cloves" widely used in the kitchen. The essential oil is obtained by distillation of cloves. After this process, a straw yellow liquid with a strongly aromatic scent will be obtained.

Cloves were a widespread remedy in the East for their digestive, tonic, antiseptic and anti-inflammatory virtues. In China it was customary to chew some to disinfect the oral cavity and purify the breath. In the 4th-5th century it also arrived in the West, in the presence of the Pope and the ritual of blessing cloves was introduced on 24 June to coincide with the summer solstice and on the day of Saint John the Baptist, then distributed to the faithful in small white bags to promote physical and spiritual health.

Well-groomed carnations give the first harvest after 5 years, otherwise it can take even 8-10. The yield increases over time, the plant remains productive for many years, some plants still give a very good harvest at the age of 100.

1. Part used: flowers, leaves, stems.
2. Method of extraction: water and steam distillation.
3. Heart note: warm, spicy scent.

- **Aromatherapy**

Clove essential oil gives energy and vigour, courage and dynamism. Useful in chronic depression and in moments of greatest discomfort. Increases resistance to stress, stimulates reaction, acts on the central nervous system, improves intellectual performance. It is to be considered a strong energy activator as it stimulates positive thinking and leads to optimism, it is a real injection of vitality. Clove essential oil is a great aphrodisiac, with warm and persuasive qualities, capable of opening each one of us to sensuality and the relationship with our partner. It strongly charges any environment with energy, freeing it from microbial and negative infestations. The result is a pleasant context in which one feels enveloped and protected and where our rational barriers are lowered to make room for instinct.

- **Tonic**

It has a stimulating action through its strong, intense and spicy aroma. Counteracts mental tiredness, drowsiness, difficulty concentrating. It is invigorating, warms, infuses a pleasant sensation of well-being and energy.

- **Massage**

1-2 drops of essential oil in a spoonful of vegetable oil to be massaged on the belly in case of intestinal spasms, or on sore muscles. It emits a pleasant warmth that penetrates deeply to dissolve tensions.

- **Contraindications**

The high component of phenols in clove essential oil can cause an irritant effect on the skin and mucous membranes at low doses and hepatotoxicity at higher doses. Its use is not recommended in case of dermatitis, gastric and intestinal inflammation. To be avoided during pregnancy and while breastfeeding.

Ginger

The spicy and tasty ginger gives us ginger essential oil: invigorating and aphrodisiac, with beneficial actions on the whole body. Known for its many properties, it is useful in case of nausea, anxiety, headaches and colds. Ginger essential oil is also seen as an excellent natural remedy against cellulite. Ginger has been used in the East for thousands of years, both to flavor and flavor foods, and as a medicinal remedy for various ailments. In Thailand, compresses and poultices of ginger root are applied, pounded and mixed with other herbs, for painful joint and muscle states that are very frequent in Muay Thai environments, the art of Thai boxing.

Ginger is also used for its dynamizing and energizing power, in all conditions of weakness and physical exhaustion. In Traditional Chinese Medicine, the root is called gan-jiang and is considered an effective Yang tonic, used precisely to strengthen male energies, fire and vitality, to treat male impotence and asthenia. In Ayurvedic medicine, it is connected to the Fire element, linked to the functionality of the spleen. Even today in many Asian countries the fresh rhizome is used in states of fatigue, to relieve toothaches, rheumatic pains, colds, malaria and all those that are defined as "humid states" such as diarrhea or excess mucus. In the ancient West, the Greeks and Romans imported ginger from the Red Sea area and knew of its important medicinal properties, as well as using it as a spice. In the Middle

Ages, the legendary Hildegard abbess of Bingen, an 11th century mystic and herbalist, recommended macerating it in wine and making compresses for eye ailments or drinking a glass of ginger wine sweetened with honey to promote vitality in convalescents and in the elderly.

1. Part used: peeled and dried rhizome.
2. Method of extraction: steam distillation.
3. Base note: warm, spicy, pungent scent.

- **Tonic on the whole organism**

If inhaled, it balances energies that are not in harmony. It helps awaken and warm up the dormant senses, improves concentration and the ability to discern. At an aromatherapeutic level, the essence of ginger acts against tiredness, weakness and nervous exhaustion; gives courage and helps to react by eliminating confusion and despair. Stimulates openness towards the outside, generating new interests. On a mental level, it favors concentration and helps to dissolve psychological knots. It is an essence that gives energy and vitality.

- **Environmental diffusion**

1 drop of ginger essential oil for each square meter of the environment in which it spreads, by burner of essential oils or in radiator humidifiers.

- **Massage oil**

In 200 ml of sweet almond oil put 40 drops, massage the painful area 2-3 times a day, or the belly in case of slow digestion, in the presence of intestinal gas and diarrhea.

- **Contraindications**

No contraindications. Ginger essential oil is photosensitive and, in case of cutaneous application, exposure to the sun is not recommended for the following 12 hours. Also, since it promotes the release of bile, ginger essential oil is not recommended for those suffering from gallstones. It is recommended not to use it to reduce nausea in pregnancy and pure on the skin.

Benzoin

Known for its toning, balsamic and antioxidant properties, it is useful against anxiety, eczema and colds. Originally from Southeast Asia, especially tropical climate areas such as Laos, Vietnam, Cambodia, China, Thailand, Sumatra and Java. Oriental folk medicine already used it thousands of years ago, in particular for its antiseptic properties. According to an Indonesian legend, he was born of a young woman, transformed into a tree to help her family in her greatest misery, allowing her to get rich thanks to her repeated bloodletting. Also called Java incense or styrax, in the fifteenth century, given its rarity and its very high price, it was sent as a gift by the Arab sultans to the Venetian doges. In 1461, Pasquale Malipero, the famous apothecary of Venice, was one of the first to use it in medicinal and cosmetic preparations. Using a cleaver also called "parang", starting from the month of May and until August, small but deep incisions are made in the bark of the plant.

The tree, which has no secretion system of its own and which usually does not produce resin, due to these incisions, due to the trauma experienced, produces a dark yellowish liquid which solidifies into grains on contact with the air, called "tears". Only when this substance has hardened well can the benzoin be collected using special tools. In this way the resin production remains constant for several years.

There are two different qualities:

1. Benzoin from Siam: with brittle and angular tears, it is the most valuable variety; yellowish in color with more amber shades and a very fine smell.
2. Sumatran benzoin: more grayish and sugary looking, less valuable whose aroma is less pungent and penetrating, and the tears are coarse, reddish-gray or almond-shaped.

Benzoin is a very effective muscle relaxant: it manages to loosen muscle tension, also acting on a psychological level, it relaxes the mind, removes stress, and therefore its external use is recommended for more or less widespread massages on the body and in the preparation of aromatic baths relaxing. Its balsamic effect helps in colds, so it is also a good expectorant. Benzoin also has incredible natural antioxidant properties, so much so that it manages to slow down the process that causes creams to go bad. And at the same time, combined with some perfumes, it succeeds with its known volatility, and stops the too rapid diffusion of aromas in the air, allowing the combined perfume itself to last longer over time.

1. Part Used: Resin.
2. Extraction Method: Solvent Extraction.
3. Base note: warm, balsamic, intense, slightly vanilla smell.

- **Invigorating**

If inhaled, it has an enveloping, sensual, balancing and energizing effect: it helps to recover psychophysical energy in the event of exhaustion or convalescence; relieves anxiety and depression.

- **Invigorating bath**

10 drops in the tub water, emulsify by shaking the water vigorously, then immerse yourself for 10 minutes to stimulate blood circulation, warm up the body and thus dissolve tensions. To prevent the flu and treat colds as they arise and to soothe sore muscles.

- **Contraindications**

Benzoin essence is neither toxic nor irritant, but may cause sensitizing effects. Not recommended during pregnancy and breastfeeding.

Himalayan flowers associated with the first chakra

Himalayan Flowers directly affect the various energy levels controlled by the Chakras, removing negative feelings and stimulating positive ones. The Himalayan Flower Enhancers were identified by Tanmaya in 1990, during a stay of several months in a Himalayan valley. The term Enhancers means catalysts, because the essences are not only remedies aimed at working on negative emotions and inner states but also favor very deep processes of energy rebalancing and spiritual development to bring to light qualities buried within the person. They can be taken pure alone or diluted together with Bach flowers or other flowers. Tanmaya's first preparations involved nine combinations, seven directly connected to the plexuses, better known by the Indian name of chakra plus a general catalyst and a flower particularly suitable for children; subsequently their number multiplied with the discovery of new flowers, suitable for modulating specific emotions.

They are Flowers with a very rapid and powerful effect, unlike Bach Flowers, which are among the slowest and most delicate; this power is sometimes very useful, other times it can represent a risk of excessive action. While the Bach Flowers can be considered mainly emotional remedies, i.e. aimed at rebalancing human emotions, the Himalayan Flowers, thanks to the nature of the soil on which they grow, essentially address the spiritual dimension of man, stimulating the need for prayer, of meditation and connection with the divine that dwells in him.

Himalayan floral essences are liquid extracts that contain the energy of the flower to be administered generally orally, and can also be used in bath water, sprayed on the body or in the environment, or combined with oil for massage.

Down To Earth

It is for all those people who feel they have lost their vital energy, the will to do, joy, physical and psychic stimuli and who feel anxiety about all material things, strong fears, exhaustion, who would like to do many things, but they always postpone. When there is a blockage or a decrease in energy in the first chakra, there is a global decrease in the vitality of the person, who feels tired and fatigued even if he is not doing major physical or mental activities: other times he did more things and yet he was less tired.

Now she no longer has interests, it seems she doesn't have time to do everything or she doesn't have the strength to do it. In all this, sexual libido decreases, there are fewer stimuli, partial impotence can occur in men and refusal to have sexual intercourse in women.

It helps in cases of reduced or absent libido and in the presence of trauma and sexual disorders.

It is usually used in cases of low morale, depression, anxiety about material existence and practical life, subtle or hidden fears, effort, stasis and lack of vital drive, joy for life, desire to do. In cases of anxiety, it can give a sense of stability and concreteness, allowing you to take small steps and do things one at a time.

We get used to following the natural rhythms of life, progressing easily, not forcing rhythms and times. Down to Earth allows energy to flow through the first chakra again, increases sexual energy, vital energy, intimacy with the Earth, the joy of living. After a few days of intake, energy returns to flow freely, tiredness passes and you can do many things that previously seemed difficult.

It helps when libido is low, enhances the sexual aspect and the ability to fully experience concrete things. It reduces anxiety about material things, subtle or hidden fears, psychophysical fatigue, lack of stimuli. To be avoided if sexual stimuli are already high. The dosage of essences, pure or diluted, is two drops under the tongue several times a day.

It often happens to combine it with the following Bach flowers: Olive, Wild Rose, Honeysuckle, Hornbeam, Centaury, Agrimony, Clematis.

Californian flowers associated with the first chakra

The Californian Flowers extend the Bach Flowers.
Richard Kats and Patricia Kaminski, founders of the FES (Flower Essence Society), together with the work of other researchers have discovered more than 150 flowers since 1979. They work on more modern and current specific problems which at the time Bach lived did not they were so preponderant or they weren't talked about like today: anorexia and bulimia, sexual disorders, diseases deriving from environmental pollution. It is possible to create composite essences by combining Bach and Californian flowers, as well as essences from other flower therapy repertoires from other parts of the world. Californian flower remedies are prepared in the same simple way as Bach flowers, by placing wild flower corollas in a glass bowl filled with spring water and leaving them to infuse in the sun for a few hours. This liquid, very rich in vital force, is then filtered, diluted in brandy and used for the preparation of the so-called stock bottles (or concentrates).

The choice of essences, as with Bach flowers, is always personalized and in relation to the mood and emotions you want to rebalance. Once the remedy or remedies indicated for the personal problem have been chosen, two drops of each are poured into a small bottle with a 30 ml dropper, filled with natural mineral water and two teaspoons of brandy as a preservative.

The dosage is 4 drops 4 times a day, for a period of a few weeks or in any case until the symptoms improve or disappear.

Being a completely natural and non-toxic cure, they have no contraindications, do not cause side effects, can be combined without problems with both traditional and homeopathic medicines (of which they are considered complementary) or other flower therapy remedies.

California Pitcher

For people who tend to suffocate, despise, deny their instinctual aspect, linked to physical energies, considering it dangerous and negative. Other people, on the other hand, let themselves be overwhelmed by instinctual impulses and unreasonably dissipate a lot of energy, reducing the material aspect of life to a squalid physicality. In both cases, the floral essence helps to harmoniously integrate physical impulses with spiritual values, allowing one to fully experience the dimension proper to the human being which is physical, mental and spiritual at the same time. Therefore this remedy can be used as a harmonizer of the energies of one's three planes when one has difficulty integrating the animal drives present in man and there is an inability to exercise one's control over them. They are usually anemic, ethereal people. It is important for the human soul to learn to distinguish, but not extinguish, its relationship to the animal world.

It is indicated for people who are unable to integrate their animal side, such as instinctual desires with their sense of human individuality.

California Pitcher Plant helps balance the immense energies of astrality with instinctive desire, so that these energies can strengthen physical vitality and nourish human spirituality.

Manzanita

To accept or rediscover a good relationship with your physical body (for example during pregnancy, puberty, menopause). Useful for people who have food problems or for women who reject the female form or their own bodies. Inner sickness manifests itself as a feeling that the body is hideous and corrupt or that it has little intrinsic value compared to the spirit. The body is often extremely objectified, exploited or emptied by strictly spiritual or ascetic regimes.

Such people adopt restrictions or rituals related to food, with a tendency to bulimia or anorexia.

This rigid view often stiffens the body prematurely and can be the cause of many diseases, despite "perfect" health regimens.

Manzanita helps the individual sweeten his relationship with matter and direct his spiritual attention to the body, thus the individual comes to conceive of the body as a reliquary or temple of the spirit.

Manzanita encourages engagement with the physical world, especially with the body, and imparts the teaching that matter is dead or inferior only when it is not accepted by the consciousness of the individual.

Mountain Pride

Stimulates the courage to face the challenges we face. For those who tend to falter and draw back when faced with challenges and cannot take a stand if they believe in something.

It is an important remedy for those who seek peace at all costs, but in reality do not realize that they are living passively, instead of actively acting to achieve their goals. The ability to act on one's concept of truth is of enormous importance. Especially in the modern world, it is of fundamental urgency that the individual learns to transform feelings of dissatisfaction or disillusionment with the world into positive energy for change.

Mountain Pride endows the individual with the archetype of the spiritual warrior, the radiation of the positive masculine for both male and female individuals.

Mountain Pride is an especially important remedy for those people who confuse peace with passivity. Such individuals must learn that affirmative action is an important healing agent, not only for personal strength and soul development, but also for true world peace. With Mountain Pride the individual learns to take a stand in the world and for the world, aligning their personal identity with the forces of goodness and truth.

Rosemary

For people who are pale, low blood pressure, introverted, physically ethereal with cold hands and feet. They live a lot in the head and therefore have no roots in the earth, or they have suffered violence and reject their bodies.

Rosemary flower essence is a strong remedy that causes awakening and incarnation, it is indicated for those individuals whose incarnation is weak or problematic, especially when the higher spiritual or thought faculties fail to act adequately through the physical vehicle.

This results in a state of reduced Consciousness in the body, with a tendency towards mindlessness or forgetfulness or hypoglycemia. In particular, the energies of the individual lack warmth and fully embodied presence.

Literally, this means that the physical extremities of the body are often cold and lifeless.

On deeper levels, this lack of warmth has to do with a sense of insecurity in one's physical body. This can sometimes be attributed to a karmic disposition of the individual, who feels ambivalent about his or her incarnation and has learned to use spiritual forces outside of the material world.

Very often this disease of the soul is caused by a trauma suffered in early childhood, in which physical abuse and the stress of the environment have forced the individual to leave his body, so that he no longer believes in his connection with the physical world.

Rosemary gives these people the ability to feel comfortable and confident in their physical body. With these renewed forces, the flame of the spirit burns more brilliantly in the body and gives its light and consciousness to the physical world.

Australian flowers associated with the first chakra

The Australian Bush Flowers are today 69 plus 19 essences created by the combination of Australian Flowers and were introduced by Ian White, Australian biologist and psychologist. They are not yet well known and used in Italy by the general public, but they are highly appreciated by flower therapists and we find Australian flowers included in many herbal and homeopathic complexes. They are among the most powerful and widely used flowers after Bach Flowers, they have a very high energy, one of the highest among floral remedies. Australian Aborigines have always used Flowers to treat discomfort or emotional imbalances, as was the case in ancient Egypt, India, Asia and South America.

The dose, for both adults and children, consists of seven drops to be taken twice a day (morning and evening) under the tongue, or in a little water. The essences should be taken for about twenty days or a month, except for particularly powerful essences.

Being a completely natural and non-toxic cure, they have no contraindications, do not cause side effects, can be combined without problems with both traditional and homeopathic medicines (of which they are considered complementary) or other flower therapy remedies. You can prepare a single remedy (whose action will then be particularly "targeted", deep and fast), or mix different remedies together; in this case it is advisable not to exceed 4 or 5 essences and, if possible, try to choose flowers with similar and synergistic properties to treat a specific problem.

Australian flowers are also very effective when applied to the skin and can be added to creams, gels, massage oils, medicated ointments or diluted in bath water. For a topical treatment, the recommended quantity is about 7 drops of each chosen remedy, to be mixed in half a cup of cream; instead, 15–20 drops of each essence should be poured into the bathtub.

The duration of treatment always depends on the individual response. A positive reaction is often obtained in about two weeks and on average two months are sufficient to rebalance numerous psychophysical problems. Some particularly "powerful" flowers (such as, for example, Waratah) usually exert a very rapid action, even in a few days. Many times, after resolving an inner discomfort or conflict, other emotional imbalances can emerge, which will gradually be treated with the corresponding flowers.

Macrocarpa

It is a remedy for energy, vitality and physical stamina for exhausted, tired and depressed people. Renew enthusiasm, vitality and energy. Excellent tonic for those who need to "pick themselves up", it can be taken in a moment of great physical stress, when resistance is needed or when a difficult goal has been reached and one is so exhausted that one cannot enjoy success. Great for people recovering.

It is important not to lose sight of the fact that this exhaustion is not only physical, but also mental, because not only can the person not do, but they can't even think. The Macrocarpa is characterized by low resistance, lack of strength and vitality and vulnerability both in their immune system and in their psychic defensive ones which leave them with a low level of self-protection. Normally they accumulate a strong negative emotional energy, defeatism and a tendency to neglect the care of their person, as if they had unconsciously given up on continuing. They have a great deal of difficulty setting boundaries, but they try and go beyond their means. They believe at 60 they have the same energy as at 20; they don't know or don't want to be aware of their limits and arrive at stressful situations without understanding the stimuli that are inside them.

Waratah

It is the remedy that helps to have courage or to raise its level. For the deep despair, the loss of all hope, the inability to react to crises. The flower gives tenacity, trust, adaptability and survival. In the Waratah emotional state, the individual finds himself in a situation that he experiences as desperate and in which, in a real or imaginary form, his survival is at stake. The person feels that he lacks the ability or courage to face it and resolve the crisis in which he feels trapped. The pressure of the circumstances in which he finds himself causes him to lose the overall vision of things or to have a confused and cloudy perception, as if there were a veil that prevents him from seeing clearly.

At the same time there is uncertainty, instability and one is inclined to react inadequately to external stimuli. This remedy is used in situations of crisis, catastrophe, trauma, panic, anguish, hysteria, loss of control. To overcome emotional blocks, great challenges, to face exhaustion states with the feeling of not being able to go on or being doomed for life. It is also a useful remedy for people with suicidal ideas, behaviors or tendencies. Given the conditions treated with this remedy, it needs to work very quickly. The initial benefits are immediate and in many cases the full effects are obtained in a short time, sometimes 5 to 7 days are sufficient.

Bach flowers associated with the first chakra

Bach flowers are an alternative medicine created by the British doctor Edward Bach, born on 24 September 1886 in Moseley from a Welsh family in England. He graduated in medicine in 1912 and immediately worked in the emergency room of the university hospital where he began to be noticed for the large amount of time he devoted to patients. He was immediately critical of other doctors, who studied the disease as if it were separate from the individual, without focusing on the patients themselves.

It is well known that our emotional states have a profound influence on our well-being and health. An altered emotional state that repeats itself every day creates real dysfunctions in our body.

Ninety per cent of the causes of human disease come from planes beyond the physical, and it is on these planes that symptoms begin to manifest before the physical body shows any disturbance. If we can identify the negative moods that crop up when we get sick, we can fight the disease better and heal faster. Using floral remedies you try to influence the deeper structures from which the disease originates. Bach flowers rebalance the emotions. They address only and exclusively how we react emotionally to the vicissitudes, experiences and problems in our days. They give great serenity and peace, courage or strength, they help us feel at the fullest of our possibilities.

They can be useful in the face of an illness, not from a physical point of view but just as a mood support. The person is seen as a complete individual where emotions are a pivotal point, and not just as a physical body with symptoms. It is therefore necessary to analyze the emotional state and not the physical symptoms, based on this the suitable remedies are found. In fact subjects with identical physical problems react and live with different emotions and feelings. Bach flowers have no contraindications and do not interact with medicines.

Bach has thus divided the 38 flowers from which the remedies are drawn. The very first flowers discovered by Bach were the so-called "12 Healers", which the Welsh doctor promptly began to experiment first on himself and then on his patients; the other 26 were discovered a short time later, divided into "7 Helpers" and "19 Assistants". Dr Bach later abandoned the distinction between 'Healers', 'Helpers' and 'Assistants' as superfluous, but many people around the world still use it. Bach Flowers do not help to repress negative attitudes, but transform them into their positive side. The Bach Flowers associated with the first chakra are only in general, because the flowers must still be chosen based on the emotion that is not in harmony and must be balanced.

Aspen

It belongs to the category of "Assistants".

Who needs this flower is a person very sensitive to negative energies, usually transmitted from the outside. They are people terrified of something that might happen, but can't pinpoint exactly what.

These fears of dark origin haunt them day and night and they can't even talk about it with others. They can't rationalize what scares them, causing apprehension, restlessness and anguish. Ghosts haunt them never allowing these people to relax.

- Symptoms: Vague and unspecified fears: the life of those who have fears of unknown origin is directed by dark and unknown forces, over which they have no control; the person lives in perennial anguish, sometimes even terrifying, and is unable to adapt to reality, clouded by the ghosts of this fearful obsession.

- State of mind: Fear. Aspen is for all undefined and vague fears; that of the dark, of magic, of monsters. Suitable for all people who have a particular sensitivity.

- Goal: Ability to understand the unknown and accept it. The floral remedy immediately stops the fantasy generated by fear, calms the person giving them optimism, makes them understand that fear was only the fruit of the mind. With Aspen your sensitivity becomes a source of security, you increase your courage.

Beech

It belongs to the category of "Assistants".

Whoever needs this flower is an intolerant and hypercritical person, he can't find anything good in his life, he also notices defects in everything and everyone to the point that nobody and nothing is ever right, thus finding himself very alone; his observation ability is above the norm finding negativity in everything around him, nothing escapes him. On the other hand, I am unable to see any flaws in itself.

- Symptoms: Excessive critical sense: the evaluation of facts, people and things is taken to exasperation; from the point of view of the "critic" nothing can ever go well. Intolerance; the lack of tolerance does not admit that others may have a different opinion. The intolerant is closed in a rigid and resentful hostility towards others.

- State of mind: Excessive care for others.

- Objective: Indulgence and tolerance. The flower remedy calms the desire to criticize and increases the level of tolerance. With Beech you accept the points of view and tastes of others with ease and understanding.

Chestnut Bud

It belongs to the category of "Assistants".

Those who need this flower take longer than others to learn life's lessons. The person with this disposition easily gets excited about any novelty or a new project, but almost never completes any idea or desire, always leaving everything unfinished. In fact, he starts a job and gets stuck halfway through and immediately starts another one, this attitude can be seen even in small things, such as books started and never finished, always repeating the same mistakes.

- Symptoms: Lack of observation skills: lack of the necessary attention intended to obtain a complete and detailed view to make a judgment or undertake something. Repetition of the same mistakes: the same mistakes are repeated for superficiality, for not having learned from previous experiences.
- State of mind: Insufficient interest in the present.
- Objective: Attention and reflection, understanding mistakes and learning from one's own experience and that of others. With Chestnut Bud every life occasion becomes a source of learning and growth. You are free from old limiting patterns.

Chicory

It belongs to the category of "Healers".

Whoever needs this flower is a person who dedicates his mental and physical strength to the needs of the people he loves, exercising a certain amount of control.

Usually the person with this nature is easily recognized because he always has something to fix for the loved one: such as the collar of the shirt, the hair, the make-up, he also gives advice on clothing, on the partner, on friendships, and asks that it be reciprocated , as if it were a job, an assembly line I give to you, you give to me. They are people who care about others to the point of being intrusive. They always find something that doesn't fit and they want to fix it the way they say, and want to. Classic interested manipulator character who probably won't easily accept this definition. But if you often think: after everything I've done, look how he treats me.

- Symptoms: Being possessive, tendency to dominate and overwhelm others in emotional relationships. Excessive concern for others, meddling and intrusiveness in the affairs of others, whether requested or not. Self pity, self compassion.

- State of mind: Excessive care for others.

- Objective: To give without asking for anything in return, respect for the freedom of others. The flower remedy will help them understand that everyone has their own destiny to follow and that there is no need to manipulate; he will also learn to give love, without expecting anything in return. With Chicory you understand the true qualities of love. You give protection and security to others in complete autonomy.

.

Crab apple

It belongs to the category of "Assistants".

Who needs this flower is a person who believes they are not completely clean, as if they wanted to drive some poison out of her body, an evil that has now been generated, or that she thinks she has. Also suitable for all those who do not accept themselves. The sensations experienced can be transformed into real phobias: phobia of any physical relationship, even a simple handshake, phobia of cleaning, phobia of insects. With Crab Apple it's easier to accept yourself for who you are, valuing our positive aspects more without remaining anchored to just the physical aspect.

- Symptoms: Feeling of impurity and dirt; the feeling of dirt is not only of a physical nature, but also mental: feeling dirty, like having something in itself that is not defined, unworthy, which can be a reason for disgust or repulsion. Shame; it is a deep and bitter disturbance when one realizes that one has acted, thought or has something reprehensible and dishonorable in oneself.

- Mood: Discouragement, despair.

- Objective: Inner purity, balance and self-acceptance. The floral remedy helps to alleviate phobias about dirt and contact with things that do not belong in your home environment: the fear that you could endanger your health will disappear and you will be able to stay in contact even with apparently not very clean people .

Elm

People who are normally strong, capable of following their vocation can go through periods of tiredness and depression and experience a feeling of helplessness and incapacity in the face of commitments beyond their real possibilities. Temporary insecurity, discouragement due to too many responsibilities, one no longer feels up to the situation, tiredness. In doing so, real energy collapses occur resulting in severe headaches, dizziness, feeling of dizziness, sweating and in extreme cases panic attacks or fainting occur.

Once the energy reserve is finished, therefore, it collapses.

- Symptoms: Inadequacy to commitments: if one comes up against a problem and cannot overcome it, a feeling of incapacity may arise and not feel up to the situation; but there are problems that are objectively beyond one's capabilities. Temporary discouragement: it is a state of mind that arises in the face of the futility of efforts undertaken and failures.

- State of mind: Discouragement, despair.

- Objective: Self-confidence, acceptance of one's limits. Elm is particularly suitable when we feel too pressured by situations or responsibilities and think that there are just too many. The floral remedy immediately gives energy, restores self-confidence in times of excessive stress, allows you not to let yourself be discouraged by the great goals to be achieved.

Mustard

It belongs to the category of "Assistants".

Who needs this flower is a person who spends moments of life in melancholy or in total despair for no apparent reason, isolates himself from everyone because it is difficult for him to hide this state of mind. Usually he spends his life very seriously and sometimes he doesn't experience the emotion because he is afraid of suffering, thus creating an emotional block; it's as if in that moment, that is when the bad event occurs, he doesn't feel the suffering because he takes life as it comes.

- Symptoms: Melancholy; it is a mood of vague sadness, accompanied by feelings of unease and disappointment. Depression, reduction of activity, slowing down of gestures, in an effort of vital economy. Despondency, despondency and prostration.
- State of mind: Insufficient interest in the present
- Objective: Joy of life and inner serenity. With Mustard the values of serenity are rediscovered and changes are accepted with the certainty of reaching the goal. The flower remedy acts immediately, the person regains serenity and then fails to give an explanation of what happened.

Olive

It belongs to the "Aid" category.

Whoever needs this flower is an exhausted person, without physical or mental energy, with every slightest effort he gets tired even with the most banal one, like brushing his teeth, combing his hair, getting dressed, reading a book, taking a walk, in short, everything becomes an insurmountable difficulty. The person is absent and without desires, from time to time a light of desire to do is turned on, but immediately loses hope because above all the physical energy fails.

- Symptoms: Exhaustion, general state indicating abnormal fatigue.
- State of mind: Insufficient interest in the present.
- Objective: Joy of life and inner serenity. Olive brings enough energy to recover all that can be recovered. Olive restores energy in an incredible way.

Rock water

It belongs to the "Aid" category.

It is the only Bach remedy that is not a flower. It must be water from an uncontaminated source, placed among plants and fields and open to sunlight. Whoever needs this flower is a very strict person in his way of life, he denies himself many entertainments and pleasures in life, respecting hard and strict rules. He thinks above all about health, he wants to be strong, active, and does everything to stay that way, he wants to be a good example for others. He is the fanatic of himself, he does not indulge in pleasures and adheres to his ideals with strength, determination and above all rigidity.

- Symptoms: Mental rigidity, excessive severity and inflexibility in the face of life rules. Poor intellectual and moral ductility. Excessive demands on oneself, demanding too much of oneself. Intolerance; the inability to accept the actions and words of others, intolerance dictated by an excessively personal vision.
- State of mind: Excessive care for others.
- Objective: Tolerance. Learn to have fun. The Rock Water remedy does not prevent people from having high ideals and trying to reach them, but it helps to limit excesses, have more flexibility and not be so intransigent with oneself.

Willow

It belongs to the category of "Assistants".

Who needs this flower is a person who has suffered an injustice, is embittered by some bad event that has happened or some project that has not been successful. The person becomes suspicious and embittered, he thinks he has been wronged by life that he cannot overcome, but in doing so there are many reactions such as swallowing anger, harboring a sense of revenge, feeling bitterness, resentment, accumulating nervousness, all without ever be able to let off steam somehow. He does not feel sufficiently rewarded and loved by life, despite the efforts. It is thought that others have been more repaid for what they have done.

- Symptoms: Inability to resign oneself to adversity: any hitch is seen as an adversity and the feeling of being treated unfairly by life becomes a certainty. Resentment: it is an attitude of aversion and animosity, as a reaction of one's sensitivity or susceptibility, to the behavior or action of others or to an external fact deemed unfair.
- State of mind: Discouragement, despair.
- Objective: Optimism in the face of adversity and a positive attitude. With Willow you are the architects of your own fortune, you feel protected and helped in achieving the right merits.

Number of the first chakra

The number connected to the first chakra is four, like the four petals of the lotus that represents it.

This number contains the very essence of Muladhara. It symbolizes stability, earthly existence, physical reality and universal manifestation. There are four directions, the phases of man's life, the phases of the moon. The number Four is the most perfect of numbers being the root of other numbers and of all things. It represents the first mathematical power, and the generative virtue from which all combinations derive. The number Four is the emblem of motion and infinity, representing both the corporeal, the sensible, and the incorporeal. The Four can be broken down into 1 + 3, the monad (the one) and the Triangle, and symbolizes the Eternal, and man who carries within himself the divine principle. The quaternary was the symbol used by Pythagoras to communicate to his disciples the ineffable name of God, which for him meant the origin of all that exists.

It is in the quaternary that the first solid figure is found, the universal symbol of immortality, namely the Pyramid. According to Pythagoras, the indeterminate dyad derived from the monad, from their union all the numbers, from the numbers the points, from the points the lines, from the lines the surface, from this the solids, of which the elements are four: Fire, Water , the Air and the Earth; and from the solids the bodies, the Decade or the Universe. Four is considered by symbology the number of reality and concreteness, of solids as well as of physical laws, logic and reason.

The Four as a manifestation of what is concrete, immutable and permanent has its geometric expression in the Square, which renders all its characteristics well. It is the number of matter; the 4 elements of earth fire, water, earth, air, concreteness, order, orientation, the cosmic cross brings together the solar points of the horizon, north, south, east, west.

Four commands the elements of the earth.

Differently from the numbers One, Two and Three, the Four, acting on a practical level, educates us to use our aptitudes to be able to realize and express what is most manifest and solid in us.

- The person characterized by the number Four is regular, habitual, responsible, traditionalist, intelligent and reserved, tenacious, never loses control of himself. If he loses his freedom he becomes self-centered, aggressive, material, limited in judgment, not very open to new things, skeptical, heavy, rigid, melancholy. The number Four is the representation of the practical sense, of concreteness, and of the constructiveness of ideas understood in a tangible sense. If one is under the influence of Four, one is prompted to act in the knowledge that one belongs to and operates in a material world. Those characterized by the Four tend to live everyday life and actively involve other people in well-defined social contexts. The Four is generally conservative and stimulates to be responsible towards the cycles of nature and to have respect for traditions. He is successful as an earth scientist, real estate developer, lawyer, administrator, office clerk, factory worker, craftsman.

Affinity with other numbers:
- Fair: 1, 2, 6 and 8.
- Excellent: 4, 7 and 9.

We can associate each number with a planet, a zodiac sign and a fundamental element of life on Earth. For Number 4 we have:
- Moon sign
- Planet Cancer
- Water element

The number 4 represents effort, renunciation, stability, the ability to carry out what one sets oneself. He never rests on his laurels, nothing comes easy to him, but he has tremendous willpower. Who is characterized by the number 4 is a person often linked to the security of the home, of affections and of the material, concrete, pragmatic, reliable. Satisfaction must be sought in the little things in life.
- The archetype of the number 4 is the Builder.
- His Shadow Number is the Prisoner.

The Prisoner represents the shadow side of the Builder and distinguishes practical and strong-willed individuals, who, however, in their identification with the Archetype, oscillate between the opposing tendencies of loyalty and determination, laziness and intolerance.

- The challenge: to develop trust in existence.

The fulcrum of this challenge is centered on the need of the subject to create stability and security around himself, without however barricading himself within rigid and obsolete mental schemes. What the Prisoner must recognize is his need to create a solidity in his life that gives him security but should not become fossilized in rigid mental schemes. The number 4 is connected to the material needs of life but the Shadow of him makes it a manic need, he lives in the anxiety of never having enough to live and he never savors and is never grateful for the goals achieved.

He tends to exaggerate any problem that becomes a tragedy for him, whether it's a health or financial problem, whether it's work or family. Furthermore, he hates changes, any variation generates apprehension and for this reason he risks remaining a prisoner, in situations that no longer have prospects for development or in relationships that are now dull and worn out. The basic problem is his family roots which have not been able to infuse him with the necessary inner security and which can go back to his childhood. Becoming aware of one's own behaviors and how far they differ from the mechanisms inherent in life, where the flow with it in its mutability is life and immobilism is non-life, can help to free the prisoner from the limits that he has self-imposed. Grounding and meditation can be excellent healing practices but, as in all cases, self-awareness is the starting point.

Phisical exercises

- **Exercise 1**

Relax the body, shake your arms and legs, sit on the floor with your back straight and then carry out alternate breathing for a few minutes, basically close one of your nostrils with the opposite hand (right nostril and left hand and vice versa), inhale gently the air, also close the other nostril by holding your breath, open the other nostril by closing the first one with the opposite hand and exhale.
Close both nostrils again and hold the breath with empty lungs and then start the cycle again.

- **Exercise 2**

Assume the quadruped position and perform the "horse's back / arched back of the cat" exercise 7 times.

- **Exercise 3**

Spread your legs shoulder-width apart, toes pointing slightly outward. From this position slowly squat down carefully keeping your spine straight at all times. Bring the upper part of the arms to the knees keeping them relaxed, always trying to make the soles of the feet adhere completely to the ground.

Do not push the limit of your reach. At the beginning it is sufficient that the buttocks are at knee height.

Inhale and exhale in this position 7 times.

Bring the sphincter up slightly each time you inhale, relax it each time you exhale, then slowly return to position.

- **Exercise 4**

Sit cross-legged with a straight back.

Rest the backs of your hands on your knees and form a circle with the thumb and forefinger of each hand, keeping the other fingers extended and relaxed.

Inhale deeply through your nose and each time you exhale sound the mantra "lam", then inhale again through your nose.

Repeat everything 7 times and during the exercise concentrate on the first chakra.

- **Exercise 5**

Lie on your back and close your eyes.

Feel how the earth supports you.

Place your hands on the lower abdomen (in the groin region) with the thumbs at pubic height and the other fingers pointing downwards.

Inhaling visualize the vital energy you absorbed, exhaling deeply let the energy flow into the root chakra. During the exercise imagine that a warm luminous stream of red color flows from your hands to the lower abdomen, create in your mind the image of the soft light flowing throughout the lower abdomen.

During the visualization inhale and exhale for at least 7 times, finally place your hands on the ground.

- **Exercise 6**

This exercise stretches the hamstrings in the back of your legs and can help unblock the first chakra, increasing flexibility in your legs. Contracted muscles denote a sense of insecurity and instability which can lead to nervousness, anxiety and fear. Keep your abdominal muscles actively engaged throughout to help support your lower back. Hold this position for 20 to 30 seconds, then slowly return to a standing position.

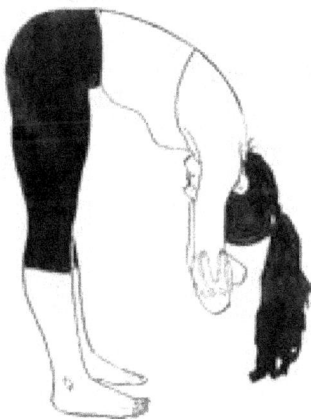

- **Exercise 7**

Spread your legs wide, placing your feet in the position that offers you the greatest stability.

Bend your knees as far as you can (over time you should be able to lower yourself so that your buttocks are level with your knees).

Come back to a standing position, then lower yourself down again.

Repeat this movement several times.

Now add a further movement: decisively throw your pelvis forward, then push it back.

Emphasize forward movement.

Perform the double motion three times as you bend at the knees.

Stay with your knees bent and repeat three more times, and finally three more times as you return to a standing position.

The most important part of this exercise is the movements of the pelvis while having the legs bent.

Repeat the complete exercise at least three times.

Stones for the 1st Chakra

In crystallotherapy stones of the 1st Chakra are considered those of black or dark color, of any type of brightness or transparency. The placement areas of the stones are: center of the pubic bone, legs, knees and feet. The crystals that can rebalance the first chakra are Hematite, Coral, Red Jasper, Obsidian, Black Onyx, Pyrite, Ruby, Tourmaline, Garnet. You don't have to buy them all, just choose the stones you prefer or which you already have.

Hematite

"Stone of Mental Domain".
Hematite owes its name to the Greek word "haimatites" which means "blood-like", as the water used when processing the hematite mineral turns a blood red colour. The custom among the Roman legions was to crush the hematite and rub the powder on the bodies, believing that this would give courage, strength and invulnerability in battle.
It's an excellent rooting stone, it strengthens the body and improves resistance to emotional stress; it is a powerful stone that helps to endure the trials and vicissitudes of life.

- It has a primarily physical and immediate effect and subsequently mental and spiritual. It dissolves and protects from negativity, transforming it into Love. It strengthens memory and attention and dissolves the mental state of confusion and indecision. It gives confidence and increases self-esteem.

It also provides a certain degree of aggression-combativeness and gives courage against injustices by venting anger in a loyal and constructive way with self-control, absorbing excessive energies of a neurotic or angry nature.
It helps in creating peace, love and kind relationships.

It creates mental organization and concentration and will help us in logical thinking and mathematics. It can stimulate iron absorption and improve oxygen supply to the body, normalizing blood pressure and body weight.

The properties of hematite to reflect any negativity where it came from are known to magicians and exorcists. Gives reliable protection against the evil eye and black magic. Used together with black tourmaline and shungite, hematite protects against geopathic stress and electromagnetic smog, as well as negativity, psychic attacks and ritual magic, returning what was sent back to the sender.

It rebalances the poorly nourished energy areas by re-establishing the right flow of energy.

It is tonic and stimulates blood circulation also helping the filtration-purification of the kidneys. It helps heal anemia, bleeding and facilitates healing, soothes joint pain and leg cramps, fights abscesses, burns, varicose veins, states of stress.

Coral

"Love and harmony".

Coral, as we know, is not part of the mineral world. Coral, in fact, is made up of communities of small polyps which form, at the base of their soft body, a calcium carbonate skeleton with a protective and supportive function. Since time immemorial, man has been looking for this marine gem as a symbol of beauty and a source of regenerating energy.

Characteristic or psychological problems disappear with the help of Coral, so that our life opens up to more collaborative and fulfilling experiences, where communication is not difficult and anxieties, suspicions and shyness appear further away and less limiting. Coral hardens the entire skeletal system and the body in general.

It exists in black, pink, red, white, blue (rare) variants. It gives off exceptional vibrations and in crystallotherapy it is linked to blood. Forms an energy shield that protects against negativity in general and some people. Associated with Turquoise it gives even more powerful protection as together they symbolize the four Elements. Stimulates energy exchange, making new energy (Prana) flow in place of the old one. It is relaxing and eliminates melancholy and worries. Strengthens personality and stimulates intuition. It awakens the stimulus and sexual attraction. Against nightmares. It is curative for many internal and external ailments. Indicated for anemia, ulcer, constipation, inappetence, indigestion, obesity, asthma, cough, lowers fever, eye and spleen problems, stimulates the secretion of mucous membranes and bile, antihemorrhagic and healing, strengthens the heart and circulation (blood cells red), removes toxins, relieves arthritic pain, regulates the menstrual cycle.

Particularly:

- Red Coral is indicated for the vertebral column, herniated discs, osteoporosis, joint blockages, stimulates blood constitution, strengthens muscles, activates the thyroid and metabolism, fights stiff neck.
- Pink Coral instills good humour, regulates the functions of the pancreas and liver, the spleen, the thymus, the symphatic system.
- White and/or Blue Coral is useful for problems relating to nerve and brain tissue and as a bone tonic (white).
- Black Coral stimulates an essential distrust in those who are too naive towards others, helps when one feels betrayed or exploited, increases attention span and learning.

Red jasper

"The Supreme Nurturer".
Jasper, in all its variants, is a unique stone that removes all negative energy present in the human body. Red Jasper is the most powerful variety. Highly prized by shamans as a sacred and powerful protective and grounding stone. In the early Middle Ages it was said that Red Jasper could give the wearer, together with God's help, the power to heal from madness and to heal if possessed by demons. According to the Bible, Red Jasper was a direct gift from God and would be the foundation stone of the New Jerusalem.

Enhances instinctive intuition and inner guidance. It supports the wearer and supports them during times of greatest stress, bringing a sense of tranquility and wholeness.

It is also a stone of deep personal fairness and justice, strengthening accountability, better choices for our evolution, and compassion.

It can have a stabilizing effect, and can help regain all of one's energy and help us use it in a more balanced way. Red Jasper aids in all critical survival areas, and of course, is an excellent stone of protection.

It brings balance, calm, courage, will, tenacity, faith in ideals and a pinch of combativeness, as for Hematite.

In the Saga of the Nibelungs it is said that a red jasper was set in Siegfried's sword. Provides security in meditation and astral travel. Brings the energy of the sun to rejuvenate and strengthen the body, making unsuspected resources available.

- Green jasper helps tissue regeneration and smell, is detoxifying and anti-inflammatory.
- Red jasper is hematopoietic and tonic (blood formation), also intervening in the re-oxygenation of the blood, acting in neurovegetative and metabolism disorders. Yellow activates the endocrine-immune system and acts on the intestine, stomach, bladder, kidneys, gallbladder, liver and bile, fights nausea.

Obsidian

"The Protector".
Obsidian is a volcanic glass that forms as a result of the rapid cooling of lava. It is found in various places in the world and in as many types, as well as in different colors. Among the many shades, there is the rainbow-colored stone, with a colorful appearance with the presence of green, purple, brown and blue. Obsidian owes its term to the Latin "obsidianus," after the Roman explorer "Obsius" who brought it to Rome from Ethiopia. The Mayans used polished obsidian as a "magic mirror," a divining tool. Obsidian stone, aligns the will with the Divine and is a powerful and protective stone to clear away negative energies. It is a very ancient stone of worship and was attributed the power to cast out demons. Another type is snowflake obsidian, which is a black and white stone. The latter has a strong spiritual vibration and psychic protection.
Obsidian has the extraordinary and unnerving ability to dig deep into its own shadows, bringing forth great intuition and knowledge, both personal and about material things. It is an effective stone for combating stress and depression, the release of old grievances and acceptance of the past. Relieves pain and stimulates blood circulation. Also, it is a protective stone against future problems.

It can especially help those who, in some way, frequently get into trouble through lack of judgment or personal bias.

Minerals vibrate especially within the base chakra and help to get rid of excess energy through the earth chakra.

In crystal therapy, obsidian helps spiritual communication, so much so that for centuries shamans have used these crystals to get in touch with their spirit guides. Furthermore, the mineral is known to amplify mediumistic powers and the gift of prophecy. Transform energy and emotions in a very powerful way. It is also a powerful grounding stone. Surrounds the wearer with an energy shield that blocks negativity. The user is provided with infinite benevolence and healing energy. Indicated to be able to discover the dark sides of one's personality in order to modify them; indicated in case of traumas, blocks, shocks and fears, as it manages to instill the energy necessary to overcome them. It can cause nightmares, due to its powerful immersion work in the unconscious world. Beneficial against pain, tension and energy blockages, stimulates circulation, tissue regeneration, heats.

Pyrite

Pyrite owes its term from the Greek "pyros" literally "fire", given the formation of sparks when it is hit. The French call pyrite "Pierre de Santé", which means "stone of health", given the strong belief already before the Middle Ages of its positive effects on health in general. Pyrite, given its resemblance to gold, has made it a strong traditional symbol in all latitudes and cultures of the world to attract money and good luck. Furthermore, pyrite symbolizes the warmth and the vital and lasting presence of the sun, favoring the recall of beautiful memories of love and friendship. It has the property of capturing earth and fire energies and this makes it an excellent tool both for balancing the root chakra and for balancing and strengthening the Aura.

Pyrite can help by giving a feeling of increased vitality during times of hard work or increased stress. It can increase physical stamina, stimulate the intellect, and help transform thought into intelligent action.

Strongly recommended for people who grapple with big conceptual ideas on a daily basis, whether in business, the arts, or education. Its properties strengthen mental abilities and awareness of higher forms of knowledge.

It can improve communication skills by driving away anxiety and frustration. Creative and intuitive impulses can be more stimulated when used together with fluorite and calcite.

It helps to make evident all the characteristics of one's personality, even the most hidden ones, allowing awareness of one's real nature and favoring openness and loyalty in relationships with other people. Counteracts anxiety and depression. It allows the causes that gave rise to a psychosomatic illness to resurface to consciousness and therefore helps to restore the healing process.

It's a pain reliever, but it shouldn't be kept too much in contact with the skin as perspiration can cause the Stone to release iron sulphide which irritates the epidermis. It is beneficial for the circulation and the respiratory system: bronchitis, tonsillitis, laryngitis, pharyngitis, tracheitis.

Black onyx

Black onyx helps to better understand the wishes of others. It therefore opens up to comparison with people and ourselves. In fact, the ear is not only stretched outwards, but also inwards. Recommended for those people who need to clarify both the goals to be achieved and the feelings in this particular moment of life. Black onyx helps to feel less the weight of other people's judgement. Thanks to this stone the will is refined and the desire to achieve the goal becomes much stronger.

Black onyx is a very powerful stone because it manages to increase fortitude. Help drive away unconstructive judgments by focusing only on what is really useful. Strengthens energetic roots and helps one find one's purpose here on earth. It is absolutely not recommended to sleep in contact with this stone. Despite being a beneficial stone, night contact is not favorable because it tends to act too "aggressive". For the night it is good to use something like rock crystal, selenite or fluorite. The black onyx must always be in the lower part of the body. So yes to anklets and bracelets. Even keeping them in your pocket is more than enough. There is a reason of course. Black aligns well with the lower chakras, should ideally not be used anywhere above the navel. The upper chakras have much more spiritual energies and do not match the earthly ones of black onyx.

Tourmaline

Red tourmaline is connected to the first chakra and is activated by the sun. Balances the functionality of the reproductive organs. Strengthens the will, passion, initiative and courage.

Black tourmaline connects to the 1st chakra and is enhanced by the indirect rays of the sun. Promotes the resolution of problems related to the bone system. It is perfect on the coccyx to relieve arthritis disorders. It is said to protect against negativity and not only in a metaphorical sense, as it is known that tourmaline is a purification stone that has the power to divert and transform negative energy, (especially that generated by electric and magnetic fields and radiation), and is therefore very protective and widely used as a grounding stone.

A rod of black tourmaline keeps company and "shield" to those who spend many hours in front of the computer or working with machinery that emits toxic radiation. These are "transparent energies" and invisible until they harm us in the physical body. It acts above all as a protective shield that defends against both negative emotions and external negative energies: it deflects them, rather than absorbing them. Carrying or wearing a piece of black tourmaline drastically reduces neurotic tendencies.

- It is one of the best stones to use when trying to ground spiritual energies, an ideal stone to place on the lower chakras in crystal therapy so as to draw energies from the higher chakras into the physical body.

Garnet

The garnet is connected to the 1st chakra and recharges in the sun.

Revitalizes the reproductive and sexual system, stimulates eroticism and passion. Gives energy to the blood. Strengthens, purifies, vitalizes the body systems, especially the vascular system; balances thyroid disorders; stimulates the pituitary gland; heals skin ailments, especially inflammations. Particularly the Eastern belief that the garnet holds not only the power to protect its user from negative energies manifested by others, but to repel these negative energies to those who originated them. Garnet can therefore be useful for total body and soul shielding.

Garnet in general enhances the imagination, helps to get out of the state of passivity and channel creative energy. It is of great help in balancing the energy system:

- Stimulates desires and lifts depressed mood.
- Develop awareness.
- Gives calm, courage, willpower.
- Does not act sedatively, but gives greater serenity, security, determination and intensity in action.

As a stone of moderation it can be used to balance the sacral chakra and excessive sexual desire and to promote the controlled growth of the Kundalini, inspiring love and passion, devotion and loyalty but also constancy in friendships. When garnet is used in conjunction with ametrine or kyanite, it can help provide past life information.

Peculiarity of the garnet is the calming of internal and non-manifest anger, which one has towards oneself.

Ruby

Revered in multiple cultures throughout history, the ruby has always been seen as a talisman of passion, protection and prosperity. It symbolizes the sun and its bright color is like an unquenchable flame. This beautiful crystal emits a pure red ray, with a vitality unmatched in the mineral kingdom.

Actively stimulates the base chakra, increasing vitality and "chi" – life force energy – throughout the body and spirit. It promotes mental clarity, concentration and motivation and gives a sense of power to the wearer, with a self-esteem and determination that overcome shyness and push to dare. The mineral encourages sensual pleasure, stimulates the heart and improves blood circulation. By precisely increasing the sexual desire, it can be used to activate the Kundalini. It has always been associated with passionate love and, in ancient times, it was considered a suitable wedding stone. The star ruby variety has the same metaphysical properties as ruby, but with greater healing power and magical energies.

It is most powerful at a full moon.

It is extremely effective in cases of self-injurious people, with erotic problems and with traumas of a sexual nature. Wearing a ruby, or carrying it with you, helps overcome tiredness and lethargy. Stimulates circulation, to regenerate the body's vitality and energy.

Those who are very nervous or irritable, however, may find this stone hyper-stimulating, thus seeing their hyperactivity increased.

Considered a blood-related mineral, it strengthens the heart, myocardium, ventricles and coronary arteries, stimulating blood circulation. It also regulates the menstrual cycle and relieves related discomfort.

Furthermore, it is indicated to detoxify the body, blood and lymph, thus helping to fight fever and infections. Stimulates the kidneys and spleen and counteracts swelling in the legs and feet. It can also help in weight regulation when it increases due to nervous hunger.

Ruby is an aphrodisiac and allows one to experience all forms of love, ranging from wild sensuality to mystical communion. It deepens the couple relationship, encouraging mutual commitment and physical and mental closeness.

It maintains the passion between two lovers and is excellent for increasing the chances of conception. It is also considered beneficial against impotence, infertility and early menopause.

It is considered, not surprisingly, a "crystal of light" in the dark moments of one's life, overcoming the overload of thoughts and stress with which the most conscientious people often weigh themselves down. It is purified and recharged on a rock crystal druze. Instead, it is better to avoid direct sunlight, which could discolor it.